EAT WHAT YOU WANT

EAT WHAT YOU WANT

*How to feel better when you
eat, without changing what
you eat!*

LUKE HASSAN, APD

Active

Active Health Clinic

CONTENTS

STEP 3: TAMING YOUR HUNGER CUES

Forward

For the past 20 years, I have consistently struggled to explain to people that it is not always what you are eating, but how you are eating it. It is from this conversation that Luke and I thought there was a huge need for people to move away from fad diets and restrictive strategies that instead of helping people, would leave people in a place of helplessness and despair.

Luke brings a unique perspective that marries together our clinical experience when helping people with invisible illnesses, especially when it is not food. The strategies in this book will help you to get a grasp on what is happening in your body, but also what you need to do to take the next steps toward choosing what YOU would like to eat, rather than your body choosing what you can eat for you.

So many people are on the hunt for the 'golden goose', that food or way of eating that makes them better or to try and 'fix' themselves, but Luke's unique stance on food and symptoms allows people to get back into their life and have more choice about their food intake. This knowledge is so valuable to me and our team and ensuring nobody that experiences these symptoms is left behind.

NATHAN BUTLER, ACCREDITED EXERCISE PHYSIOLOGIST AND FOUNDER OF ACTIVE HEALTH CLINIC, WITH OVER 20,000 HOURS OF EXPERIENCE WITH INVISIBLE ILLNESSES.

DISCLAIMER

In this book you will find a lot of practical strategies and information to help you be like Mrs G (that will make more sense in a moment) and live with freedom in your food intake again. This book is not intended as a 'diet', or to treat any medical condition, and is general advice. These strategies will help you in almost every circumstance in some way, however, I feel that it is necessary to say that there are always other reasons why people could be struggling with food and the issues outlined in this book, and I would encourage you to reach out to your healthcare team (or even myself if desired) if you have any concerns about your symptoms, or if you feel that the tools in this book have not been the right fit for you.

Take care, and happy eating!

- Luke

| 1 |

Introduction

I want to tell you a story about Mrs G. Mrs G was not 'all G' the day I met her- it was a cold and windy September day, which was fitting for Mrs G's main complaint: a whole lot of bloating, wind, and discomfort in the stomach area. This would happen after eating any meal, but particularly when she finished her dinner meal. Now before coming to see me, Mrs G tried almost every diet under the sun to get rid of her bloating. She tried cutting out carbohydrates; she tried adding more carbohydrates (why does it always have something to do with carbohydrates...?). Mrs G tried adding fibre by eating more vegetables, she tried having activated charcoal after every meal; she tried the low FODMAP diet, she tried intermittent fasting, but no changes that Mrs G made seemed to make any difference at all. What also had not changed was that Mrs G was terribly unhappy with the way that she felt after she ate. Being an Italian mother in her mid-50's, Mrs G loves food, and loves the joy and affection she can give to her family through the food she cooks. All these diets had taken their toll and Mrs G was adamant that she did not want to go on another diet that would probably end with her feeling exactly the same as she did at that first appointment. So, I levelled with Mrs G and told her that there were a few really simple tips that we could put into place, that we could treat as somewhat of an experiment, and this would mean she would have nothing to lose. I suggested that her husband (who suffered from a similar set of symptoms, she told me) could also take up the challenge, and that they could keep each other accountable to these changes, and if we just gave it a try for a couple of weeks, what would there be to lose?

Mrs G went home with just a few simple tips that you are going to learn in this book and put them into place most of the time (but not perfectly) over the next three weeks. When we came back for our follow-up appointment, things were not perfect, but they were better. I was really proud of Mrs G for putting these strategies into place and I encouraged her to continue to build on these tips, with just a few small tweaks to make them more sustainable and realistic in the long-term. Before long Mrs G reported that her bloating, particularly after dinner, had gone away completely. Mrs G said she had a spring in a step during the day again - much to my amusement (and much to her daughter's dismay) she had been up on the roof cleaning the gutters the weekend before our appointment - something Mrs G hadn't been able to do in years because of her lightheadedness and lack of energy during the day. Most important of all for Mrs G, she felt she was able to eat what she wanted without feeling unwell and that fear of feeling unwell was slowly but surely becoming a thing of the past.

If you feel like Mrs G's story resonates with you, that it doesn't seem to matter what you eat, you just always seem to feel icky afterwards: whether that looks like bloating, pain, nausea, brain fog, fatigue, or just a general feeling that food isn't doing what it's supposed to be doing.
If you've tried multiple diets or 'ways of eating' that are supposed to help with this feeling, and they just haven't - OR you don't WANT to try

some abstract and restrictive diet to try and feel better with food - this book is for you.

In 20 short pages you will learn how to:

- Stop feeling nauseous, bloated or in pain after you eat
- Feel energised from your food again
- Enjoy your favourite foods again without fear.

So, are you ready to get started with feeling better after you eat?

STEP 1: REST AND DIGEST

| 2 |

Hectic lives don't equal tummy vibes.

The pace that we move in this modern life is INSANE. The rate at which we are expected to complete tasks; to keep up with the latest in news, and pop culture, and sport, and know what people are doing in politics; what the latest social movement is, and what the latest health craze is; it is information overload at its most extreme. Not to mention that we are hit with a massive case of FOMO (fear of missing out) if we happen not to be able to keep up with all of this! While people might recognise this is contributing to the rising levels of anxiety and depression, not to mention other mental health conditions that we see prevalent in our society, people don't often link the fact that these conditions and the things we experience that preceded them actually impact our physical health as well. Our nervous system is our control centre: governing both brain and body, and therefore the way that our psychological and physiological response operates. This means that we cannot really separate our psychological stressors from our physical stressors, one will always affect the other – try living without your head, for example (actually, no, please don't!). This stress, at different times, might come from our jobs, our relationships with friends, family or a partner, the study that we're doing, or the environment that we find ourselves in that doesn't quite feel 'right'. All these situations are an example of the body, through the nervous system, potentially deciding to take over and protect. After all, our nervous systems developed in a time where we needed to be able to run away from a lion if it came to attack our camp. Even though this might not be a reality for many of us today, when we encounter environments or situations that warrant a stress response, that worry us or make us feel anxious, the physiological consequences are the same. These events result in an increased release of adrenaline and cortisol, the acute and chronic stress hormones that keep our system alert and 'on guard' in an attempt to keep us safe.

This 'pedal to the metal' attitude that we have to life is one of the primary causes of stress in our lives today. When we put a metaphorical brick on the accelerator pedal in our lives, we are likely to experience increased, unintended adrenaline and cortisol responses that keep our system wired, even in times where we are meant to be resting. Have you ever wondered why you lie awake at night, tossing and turning, thoughts running at speed through your brain, seemingly unable to relax or settle down enough, or feel safe enough from those thoughts even, to get to sleep? Or, for those of us who enjoy exercise or structured movement, and generally find it a relaxing and helpful activity - have you ever been so consumed by other events of the day that you just haven't felt like the exercise provided the release you needed? An increase in stress hormones is just one of the reasons this could be happening. Another way that this can be explained as a shift into 'fight or flight' - your nervous system being so overwhelmed - simply by the pace that you are travelling in life, that it feels the need to turn on the systems that were designed to help you flee from danger; or to stay and help you fight the danger.

Doesn't seem like a useful way to respond to the stresses of everyday life, does it? If you're familiar with the 'fight or flight' concept, you might also be familiar with the equal and opposite response, or 'rest and digest'. You can clearly see from the above description of the pace of our lives how our bodies might, by no intention of our own, fall out of that rest and digest phase into the fight or flight phase quite easily. And if you understand the metaphor of fight or flight being developed for us to be able to run away from a lion, **you will understand that the last thing we need to do when we're running away from the lion is digest our food**. So, what is another unintended consequence of our busy fast-paced hectic lives? Our body is in a state where, more often than we realise, we are not physiologically ready to accept, digest and absorb food.

ACTIONS

Let's take some practical steps to think about what may be pushing you toward flight or flight, and away from rest and digest. Identifying these factors will be the first step to getting you back on the roof, doing what you love and eating what you like, like Mrs G.

Have a look at the boxes below: what are some of the things that keep your internal accelerator flat to the floor?
- work (doing your job) and
- work (the environment that surrounds you while you work)
- study
- friendships
- relationships
- family
- food thoughts
- lack of restful activities
Other?

_____

_____

| 3 |

Learn to rest, and the digest will follow.

When you think of rest, what comes to mind? Most of us will be thinking sleep, holidays, a 15-minute power nap... These are all examples of
restorative rest. Taking an extended period away from the business of
life to just chill. But those things are not really achievable for us in the
middle of our workday, are they? This begs the question: what do we do
when we notice that our body is becoming wired, to try to settle that
stress response that we talked about in the previous chapter - and it's not
quite appropriate for us to take a nap?

Thankfully, there are other types of restorative rest, and you've probably
heard of them before. Restorative rest throughout the day is actually
needed for us to stay at peak performance. Have you ever noticed that
you're actually more productive after you've taken a break to go and get
a coffee, or have a chat with your colleague that you enjoy talking to, or
once you get over that post-eating lull after lunch? How nice would it
be to leave work for the day feeling like you still have something left in

the tank? When you take proper breaks, it's possible - this is a sign of you actually allowing your body and your brain to not constantly be in that heightened state of performance that's required for work. The fact is that your body doesn't desire being in that heightened state consistently - one of the reasons being that the body knows it's not able to digest and absorb food properly, and therefore restore its energy levels adequately, when you are consistently wired. Just like restorative rest is needed to keep us at peak performance throughout the day and help us to be as efficient as possible with our work, the same can be said of restorative rest being important for the way that our gut works.

With all this talk about rest, I can imagine what thoughts are going through your mind. "Yep, that all sounds great, but when am I supposed to find the time to do all of this resting you speak of?". What if I told you that they were already dedicated times in the day allocated for rest that are completely and totally socially acceptable, and that 95% of businesses already allow for? It would seem like some sort of a miracle, wouldn't it? Well, it's not really a miracle, but it does make it a whole lot easier for you to actually incorporate into your day.

What are these rest times I speak of?

Mealtimes!

That's right, your morning coffee break, lunchtime, and afternoon break, are all the excuse that you need to take some time to refuel your body - not only in a physical sense through consuming food, but in a holistic sense, by using that eating occasion to wind down your over-engaged brain. This, in turn, focusses your bodies' entire resources on digesting and absorbing your food.

It's a little bit more than just sitting down to eat, however. As you would be aware, we humans will multitask by default, especially when we're wired - for some reason our brains seem to think we will power through more stuff if we never take a break, but as we talked about before, we know that in reality, this just causes more overwhelm and less productivity. So if we're going to get our body to focus on one thing - that is, digesting our food properly to make sure we stop feeling icky after our meals – here are three tricks that make our physiology, as well as our psychology, fall into line.

1. Single task, where the outcome does not matter:
Multitasking kicks our brain up a gear and increases the need for blood flow away from the gut. When we're trying to eat, multitasking 'distracts' our body from the task at hand, preventing us from doing the job of digesting in the most efficient way possible. Think about it like an athlete at game time – they need to be completely focused on their role to perform to the best of their ability. If the athlete is thinking about their plans after the game, the crowd, their competitor, their chance of getting injured, the argument they had during the week... their chance of performing their best severely decreases.

It makes sense that while we're eating, we engage in an activity (if we can't just sit quietly and eat) that is a single task. We like to call this a 'green time activity' - in reference to a traffic-light like system, this task is something that facilitates restorative rest. The part where the outcome of that single task doesn't matter also relates to our level of arousal during that eating period. The best way to think of it is that if we need to engage our 'rest' to most efficiently 'digest', then we need to be as close to being physically, emotionally, and cognitively switched off as possible. This means that, while eating, there's no watching your team play footy, no overly 'emotional' conversations with the family (arguing), and, most importantly, no sitting at the desk working!

2. Sitting to promote blood flow:
When we stand and eat, centring our blood flow on our gut is made more difficult by the effect of gravity. Bringing your body closer to horizontal works to decrease that difficulty. Obviously, we don't want you to be lying down and risk choking on your meal - but if you find it's not causing other problems (read: heartburn/indigestion) a slight recline with legs elevated is the best.

3. Remember to breathe before a meal:
You might not be a big fan of breath work - I know I'm not (unless it's with a spot of gentle movement like yoga). But breath work isn't always about minutes on end of focusing on pushing your chest, then stomach, out; then sucking your stomach, then chest, in - or counting your inhale and exhale in a square. Just ten deep, diaphragmatic breaths can help to reset your nervous system and engage your rest and digest. Scan the QR code below for an example video and give it a try next time you eat!

STEP 2: THERE IS NO NEED FOR SPEED

| 4 |

The fast and the furious…
eaters.

'You are a human garbage disposal unit…' My mother used to say to me after absolutely demolishing one of my favourite meals. It must have seemed that whatever was put in front of me was almost completely gone as soon as it touched the table. That was ok when I was a teenager, and nothing seemed to affect me like it does now. I always had chronic reflux, but we just thought that was something that I would grow out of. Unfortunately, this was not the case: it only just kept getting worse and for some reason I couldn't figure out why – I felt like my symptoms were out of control. I didn't realise what was really going on until one day I sat down to a plate of my mother-in-law's Bolognese pasta. They may as well have called me a human vacuum cleaner that night because I hoovered this plate of pasta into my mouth and down my throat as fast as I think a human could possibly do it. And straight afterwards, I felt nothing. It was like I hadn't eaten anything yet. But over the course of the next 5 or 10 minutes I started to feel extremely unwell, and that all too familiar reflux came back, and I couldn't get rid of it. I was also bloated, in pain, and just felt generally gross for about an hour afterwards. Does this story sound like it could be your story? Does it make you feel uneasy to think that that could be you this afternoon, or this evening or maybe tomorrow?

Think about the way that you eat food: would you consider yourself a shoveler or a grazer? If you resonate with the story above, you will probably consider yourself a shoveler. Shovelling makes more sense as a metaphor for food intake, perhaps, than vacuuming - the thought of the literal motion of using cutlery to put food in the mouth is a nice rendition of digging a hole. As the metaphor would have it though, no one digging a hole does so with little pieces of dirt - they get as much dirt as possible on the shovel and toss it away - almost like I put away that plate of pasta.

Grazers, on the other hand, take their time with their food. They might pick at a meal slowly rather than heap food into their mouths. They are quicker to realise that they are full, but also might return to food in between meals for snacks more frequently across the day. In this way, grazers may seem more like cattle, gently nibbling away as they see necessary, all day long. After working with many shovelers and many (but not as many) grazers, one thing is clear: grazers are more content with the way that they feel after meals, both mentally and physically; they have more energy, less gut symptoms, and less body-image related concerns because they've been able to listen to their bodies NATURAL HUNGER CUES (more about that gem in the next section) to decide when they are full.

A quick note on the need for speed...

This need to eat food so quickly, often in my experience, stems from one of two things: a genuine love of the food that you are eating, and/ or a hand-me-down of food insecurity that exists because of our grandparents and then, subsequently, our parents' uncertainty around where they were getting their next meal from because of food scarcity in times of hardship, for example, wars, famines, and floods. This is also why you may feel like you need to eat everything on your plate, to not be wasteful, even if you couldn't fathom putting another morsel of food in your mouth. Most of us don't have this kind of problem anymore, but we can act like we do due to feeling pressured to fit everything, even our mealtimes, into this schedule that allows us to keep our heads above water with our crazy daily lives. We have fridges, we can store leftovers, and we don't need to give our bodies this overload that is likely contributing to the symptoms we are trying to address with this book.

In saying this, I wholeheartedly recognise that food insecurity is still a genuine issue for some people, and if that is you reading this book, please don't feel that you must go on this journey alone. Below, there is list of resources/places you can go to help you on this journey.

RESOURCES/PLACES THAT CAN HELP YOU IF YOU LIVE WITH FOOD INSE-
CURITY (Australia only)

https://askizzy.org.au/
https://www.secondbite.org/for-individuals
https://www.ozharvest.org/food/receive-food-individuals/
https://www.empoweraustralia.com.au/programs/food-relief-centre/

| 5 |

Be the tortoise.

Remember the old story about the race between the tortoise and the hare? Spoiler alert – the tortoise wins – and forever instils in listeners that slow and steady wins the race. It's safe to say that, being the winner, the tortoise felt a lot better after that race than the hare. In this chapter, I'd like to invite you to 'be the tortoise' and feel the benefits of eating your food slower.

In previous chapters, we talked about slowing down and resting around your meals, to enable your body to engage its 'rest and digest' mode and help process the food that you are consuming better. For similar reasons, we now need to talk about slowing down DURING your meals. There are more benefits to slowing down our meals that we'll talk about in step 3 of this book, but for now, let's look at some ways to stop shovelling your food, and help reduce that sickly, overfull, unwell feeling after eating.

The below three strategies are ways that patients of mine have achieved their goal of slowing down their meals. To help with de-identification (and to help you remember their strategies) I've provided each example with a handy nickname. So, without further ado, meet:

- "The New-Music Guru" - This Guru found that listening to music, and particularly finding new music that they enjoyed, was a joyful hobby that fit the criteria of a green time activity (see chapter 2: single task, outcome doesn't matter). So, to help slow them down while eating meals, they started to use the 'new music radar' playlist on their streaming service as a circuit-breaker. Every time a song finished, or they realised they didn't like the song, they would put down their cutlery/the food that they were eating (wiping their hands if necessary) and selected a new song. Here's the catch: you can't touch your phone while holding cutlery/food!

- "The Mathematician" - This Mathematician, it seems, loved maths, particularly fractions. They would divide their plate up into sections like a pie chart and would rest after each section for a dedicated period of time. In a variation of this, I've negotiated with people before that after 50% of whatever's left on their plate, they take a break for a full minute - again, the catch being that in the break, they aren't allowed to be holding their cutlery or their food. It might be a little rigid, so this strategy won't be for everyone, but it is effective.

- "The Chew Chew Train" - you might have guessed by the name, but this person would count their chews - 10 to be exact - before they would swallow their mouthful. Very tedious, for sure, but adequate chewing is one of the most important ways that the brain recognises that you're eating and starts noticing the amount of food that you are consuming, so it can tell you when to stop.

The key to all these strategies is to have a prompt for rest within the meal so that you are constantly brought back to putting your cutlery/

food down, which allows your body to catch up with how much food you've actually eaten, enabling you to monitor this and not overeat. This leads VERY nicely into:

STEP 3: TAMING YOUR HUNGER CUES

| 6 |

Respecting queues.

Imagine for a moment that you're in a queue of some sort. Perhaps it's the line to get to the self-serve checkout at the supermarket, or to order food at a takeout place. Now imagine someone having the AUDACITY to cut in front of you in that line. How do you feel? Angry? Frustrated? Offended? What are your first thoughts/actions? Is it cursing that person, calling them an ignorant so-and-so? Only someone with no thought for other people's or their own life would ever contemplate such anarchy. How dare they not respect the order and authority of the queue?

I'm being dramatic, for sure, but most people will admit that they get a mix of negative feelings when someone doesn't respect a queue. Now that I've got you thinking about this, I'd like to propose that it's not just those external QUEUE'S that cause negative internal feelings when they aren't respected.

Your body has an amazing way of letting you know what it needs, and it's super powerful. It literally sends you feelings that for some reason, you just can't seem to shake very easily. We know these as 'bodily cues', and they come for all types of things: for rest and sleep, for movement, and importantly for us, hunger and fullness. All of these cues help keep us in a state of internal balance, or 'homeostasis'. And when you don't respect these bodily cues, said body is likely to get unhappy about it, just like we would be unhappy if someone didn't respect our place in the queue.

| 7 |

Identifying your CUES.

It's important, then, that we actually know what these cues are. They will differ from person to person but do follow a consistent trend within a person, so after a little bit of searching, should be noticeable enough to identify. It is true that some people have very little hunger/ appetite cues, and these people will most likely need to create these again - but that's a topic for another book.

So, what are YOUR hunger cues? Well, these will differ from person to person, but most people will identify with at least one or two, if not more, of the following:

- 'Tight' feeling in the stomach, sometimes described as pain or a 'yearning',
- Intensifying bowel sounds,
- Decreased focus on cognitive tasks; brain fog, difficulty word-finding, engaging in multitasking or intense conversation,
- Lower tolerance to others; increased irritability, lower mood,
- Headaches,
- Sleepiness/fatigue,

- Increased thirst.

All of these sound particularly uncomfortable and frustrating - these are what we would consider to be 'shouting' messages from the body rather than a gentle nudge. For most people, the first sign of hunger is that slight discomfort in your stomach, followed by an increase in thinking about food. To prevent these more intense messages from the body listed above, it is worthwhile being mindful of those less-intense messages, tuning into them and becoming more accustomed to listening to them, so that you can quench your hunger earlier. This has three benefits; 1. You don't have to feel so overly hungry at any given time, 2. You have a more measured and consistent energy intake over the day, and **3. You don't give way to overcompensating for that increased hunger and overeat,** which could be contributing to your gut symptoms post-food consumption.

Takeaway: learn to listen to your hunger cues and gratify them EARLY.

Similarly, what are your fullness cues? These are often much harder to decipher than hunger cues because, for a lot of people (especially shovelers), they just seem to come on all at once.

Again, each person will experience these messages differently - it could simply be a feeling of not wanting to put any more food into the body - something that is subconsciously understood, rather than felt. Or, fullness cues could include feelings of content, satisfaction, a sense of re-energisation etc. On the other hand, those that don't report experiencing the above might not experience fullness cues as much as symptoms, such as bloating, pain, indigestion, nausea, or pressure in the gut. Symptoms might also include brain fog, dizziness, and/or sleepi-ness/lethargy for a certain period after eating.

Another important question is 'when do you pick up on your fullness cues?'. Do they come on in the middle/toward the end of finishing a portion of food on your plate? Is there a gradual rise in fullness, like you're filling up a petrol tank, or is it more sudden? This can often be where the problem lies when it comes to overfullness being the root cause of these gut symptoms. If we have no awareness of our fullness as it approaches a 'comfortable' capacity, it is way too easy to eat well above that mark and, subsequently, we feel rubbish.

To help with recognising both hunger and fullness cues, I've created a couple of handy resources to help you group these cues into a 'traffic-light'-style rating system, with some examples of our orange (warning) and red (stop) sensations, and space to fill in your own as you continue to explore these for yourself. I'd encourage you to use the below QR codes to download these and fill them out, so you have a tangible refer-ence that you can use to assist you with this process.

Using steps 1 and 2 above, as well as the 'traffic-light' resources below, you'll have more of an idea about your own answers to these questions now. It will take some time, some careful thought, and consideration as to what your individual cues are, as well as some practice with learning when your fullness cues in particular start approaching during a meal. Once you become more confident with these two things, however, you will find that your comfort levels after meals increase dramatically.

Here is another tip to help you with your journey to recognising your hunger. Whichever strategy you decided to take on board from step 2 (remember all the interesting names for people and their habits for slowing down their eating?), during the period that the strategy gets you to put down your cutlery/food and stop eating, ask yourself: "what is my level of fullness right now?". Be really introspective about it, and see if you can, after a while, pick the time where you need to stop eating to feel comfortable.

GREEN LIGHT
GO - CONTINUE WITHOUT FOOD

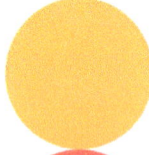

ORANGE LIGHT
WARNING: HUNGER APPROACHING

RED LIGHT
STOP: EAT NOW

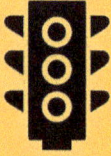

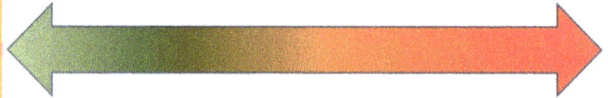

TRAFFIC LIGHTS - HUNGER

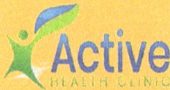

WHAT ARE MY ORANGE LIGHTS:

Ex. Decreased concentration, intensifying bowel sounds, yearning in stomach...

WHAT ARE MY RED LIGHTS:

Ex. Headache, lightheadedness, increased irritability, nausea...

WHAT ARE MY SOLUTIONS:

Ex. meal or snack?

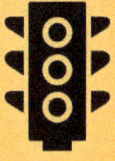

TRAFFIC LIGHTS - FULLNESS

GREEN LIGHT
GO - CONTINUE EATING

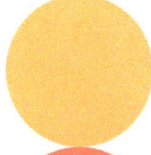

ORANGE LIGHT
WARNING: FULLNESS APPROACHING

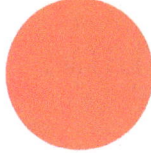

RED LIGHT
OVERFULL - STOP EATING

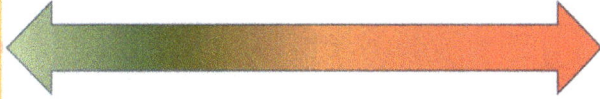

WHAT ARE MY ORANGE LIGHTS:
e.g. becoming bored of taste/texture, feeling content, nibbling

WHAT ARE MY RED LIGHTS:
e.g. bloating, pain/cramping in the gut, indigestion, nausea, reflux...

WHAT ARE MY SOLUTIONS:
What are you going to do to make sure you slow down at the orange light?

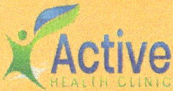

Active
HEALTH CLINIC

| 8 |

Summary.

In essence, this book comes down to one line: 'slow down and listen'. It's really hard to get a grip on what your body is trying to tell you - the messages that it has regarding your appetite - if you don't take a break from your busy life to 'check in' with yourself regularly to ensure you're feeding your body when it's asking to be fed, preventing the build-up of an appetite that is likely to lead to you shovelling down food. Additionally, slowing down before, during, and after you eat, allows you to listen to those hunger and fullness cues so that you can eat the right amount for your body. This prevents you from overfilling the system, which can result in feeling nauseous, bloated, in pain, lethargic or sluggish after you eat, and gives you confidence that you can savour your favourite foods without scoffing them down and feeling unwell because of them.

It is my hope that through the tips and strategies outlined in this book, you can prevent a descent into the world of restrictive diets, strange supplement regimes and a lower quality of life, and simply get your love of eating, and eating occasions, back to what it once was.

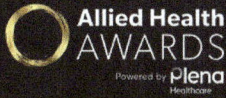

Allied Health
AWARDS
Powered by Plena
Healthcare

WINNER

2020-2021 AUSTRALIAN
ALLIED HEALTH EARLY
CAREER EXCELLENCE

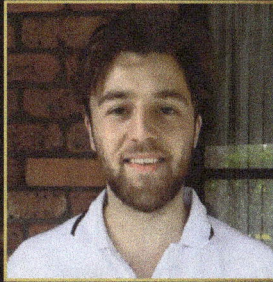

Luke Hassan

Luke was recently voted by his peers as the 2020-2021 winner of the Allied Health Early Career Excellence award, at the Australian Allied Health Awards.

If you would like more information about Active Health Clinic, just scan the QR code above!